Aubrey!

Lightning speed
Lainey Riley

June

bot :)

h h !

coach mommy/Emily

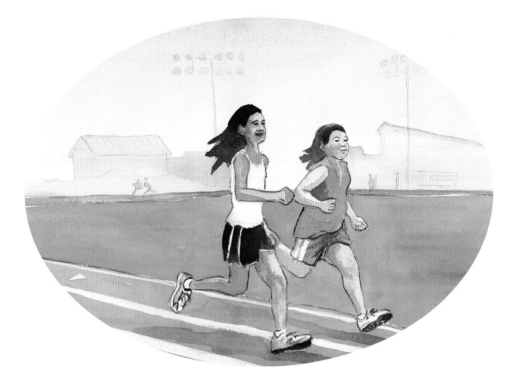

We Are Girls Who Love To Run

Somos Chicas y A Nosotras Nos Encanta Correr

By Brianna K. Grant

Illustrations by Nicholas A. Wright

Spanish translation by Ana C. Venegas

For additional information go to www.balancedsteps.com

For my family who cheers, "Go, Runner, go!" as I stride onward to reach my goals – your love
and encouragement put zing in my step. Also, for girls and women who discover the joy
and inner balance that come with the camaraderie of running.
-BKG

To Emily, whose support, understanding and love are what keep me painting and drawing.
To Makayla, Lily, and Jenna, who are the twinkles in my eye!
And finally to Mom and Dad - where would I be today without you?
- NAW

Special thanks to the following people who helped make this book possible:

Joan Stockbridge, editing (English)
Denise Hatcher, editing (Spanish)

We Are Girls Who Love To Run
Copyright 2008 by Brianna K. Grant

Illustrations copyright 2008 by Balanced Steps, LLC
All Rights Reserved.
Printed in China.
Book design by Kirk Werner
Author photo by Jim Hallas

Balanced Steps, LLC • P.O. Box 1179 • Duvall, WA 98019

or visit

www.balancedsteps.com

ISBN 978-0-9798511-1-7

Library of Congress Control Number 2007906934

The illustrations for this book were painted on 140lb Cold Pressed Arches Acid Free Watercolor Paper.

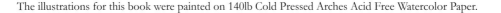

What Others Are Saying About We Are Girls Who Love To Run

"Brianna Grant's message for girls to take time to dream and stay connected with others who share their passions is one that I take to heart. Goal-setting, teamwork and celebration of successes with those who helped me are central to my own training."

— **Deena Kastor, Olympic Medalist and American Record Holder**

"Being happy isn't about being perfect, especially when it comes to eating well. Eating is about finding out what food has to offer, and striking a balance between your needs, personal preferences, culture, and family experiences. *We Are Girls Who Love to Run* addresses those important life aspects, while making the book enjoyable, personable and applicable to any girl who reads it."

— **Liz Applegate, Ph.D., Director of Sports Nutrition, UC Davis**

"*We Are Girls Who Love to Run* speaks to the whole child, acknowledging the complexities of girlhood and celebrating successes girls can discover in their own lives. Not only is the book an inspirational introduction for a group run, but also makes for a strong post-run journaling prompt."

— **Carol Goodrow, Author/Illustrator, Educator and Founding Editor, KidsRunning.Com**

"*We Are Girls Who Love to Run* captures the nurturing essence that comes with being a part of something bigger than yourself. It cheers on females who enjoy the camaraderie of working together to reach a goal, a bond that builds confidence and friendship through exercising and living a healthy lifestyle."

— **Jamie Allison, CEO and Founder, Moms in Motion**

"Brianna Grant's message of mentorship and working together is one that supports girls as they discover the value and reward of setting and achieving their goals. *We Are Girls Who Love to Run* is a book to share with friends before or after a run, helping process all of the ways that running makes you feel – strong, successful, peaceful, beautiful and loveable!"

— **Sarah Nixon, Creator and Director, Fit Girls**

"With her debut book, Brianna Grant's message bounds forth, challenging girls of all ages to get out and move past physical, emotional, and social hurdles. This inspiring message is a much needed resource in the fight against that preventable disease -- childhood obesity. These words literally make this 35 year-old girl want to get out and run."

— **Noelle Grosso, President, Running Kids**

Foreword

I am always amazed at how life offers me connections with the "right" people at the "right" time. The fact that you are reading this foreward indicates that on some level you are in the right place and at a right time to be connected to what lies before you.

Brianna Grant, author of this book, is one of those right people at the right time. Her understanding of what Girls on the Run is all about was obvious from the get-go. Her ability to articulate the "feminine side" of running has me awestruck as her words flow in a joyful stream of celebration, wonder and strength.

When Brianna approached me about writing a book for girls that captures the spirit of running, I knew that what she would create would be amazing. After reading her manuscript, I was certain she "got it"! Each time I read *We Are Girls Who Love to Run*, I am reminded of the positive and profound influence running has on not just our physical selves but our emotional and spiritual selves as well!

I invite you to celebrate the joy of running, the wonder of being a girl and the strength that comes through "daring to try" by reading this book. Feel again the vibrancy that comes with being a "girl who loves to giggle and feel the wind in my hair...a confident girl, embracing my identity and loving life."

With joy abounding, I invite you to be a *Girl Who Loves to Run*.

Molly Barker, M.S.W.
Founder and Vision Keeper
Girls on the Run International
www.girlsontherun.org

I am a girl who loves to run.

Soy una chica y me encanta correr.

Some days I run quickly, my feet carrying me like lightning racing the wind. Other days I walk, soaking in the world around me. Whether I run, stroll, or amble, the time is mine to enjoy.

Algunos días corro rápidamente y mis pies me elevan como relámpago por el viento. Otros días camino, y contemplo todo lo que sucede alrededor de mí. No me importa la velocidad, el tiempo es mío para gozar.

I am beautiful.

Soy hermosa.

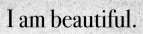

When I smile, my eyes sparkle, and my spirit glows for the world to see. Freckles parade across my face. My arms and legs are graceful as I circle the track.

Mis grandes ojos chispean cuando sonrío y reflejan a todo el mundo mi resplandor interno. Un desfile de pecas baila de una mejilla a otra por mi cara. Mis piernas y brazos se mueven graciosamente mientras corro por la pista.

I am a good friend.

Soy una amiga buena.

I love to be boisterous. My friends count on me for silly songs, laughter, and high-fives on good days. I'm a good listener, and my friends call on me for encouragement when they have bad days. I value my friends' feelings and take the time to apologize when I make mistakes.

Me encanta ser bulliciosa. Mis amigos cuentan conmigo para las canciones graciosos, para reír y para felicitarlos con una porra cuando tienen buenos días. Me gusta escucharlos y darles palabras de aliento cuando tienen malos días. Valoro los sentimientos de mis amigos. Me disculpo con ellos cuando cometo error y así les demuestro que son honestas y dignas de confianza.

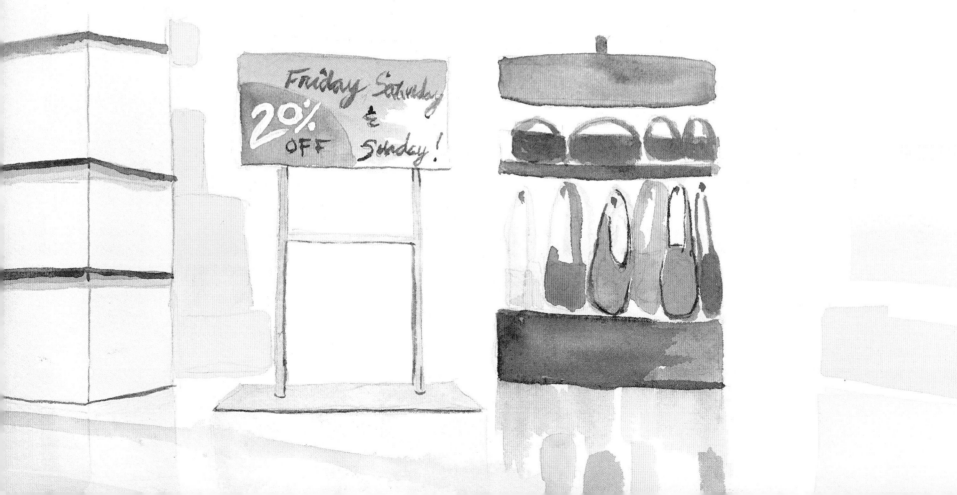

I take care of my body.

I help my mom choose colorful fruits and vegetables for after-school snacks. I sleep peacefully at night, dreaming that my swift feet are racing over hills and across meadows. My health shines out in a radiant smile.

Cuido mi cuerpo.

Ayudo a mi mamá escoger frutas y legumbres sanos y de varios colores para hacer meriendas para después de la escuela. Por las noches duermo tranquilamente mientras sueno que mis pies vuelan sobre los prados y las colinas. Mis buenos hábitos se reflejan en mi sonrisa radiante.

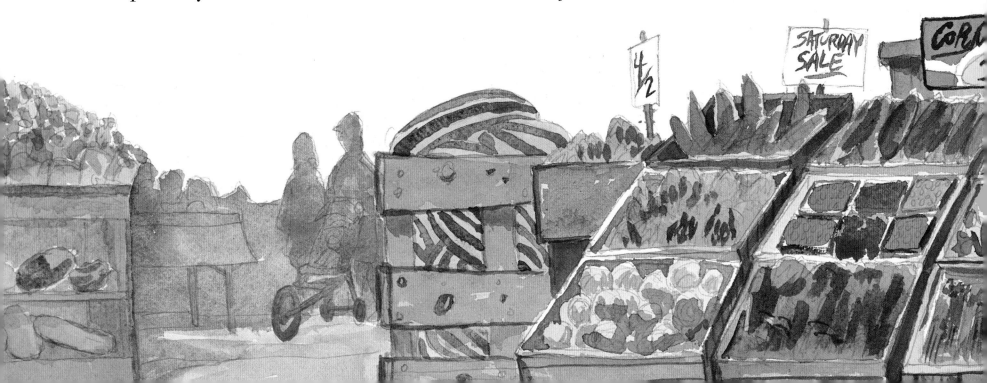

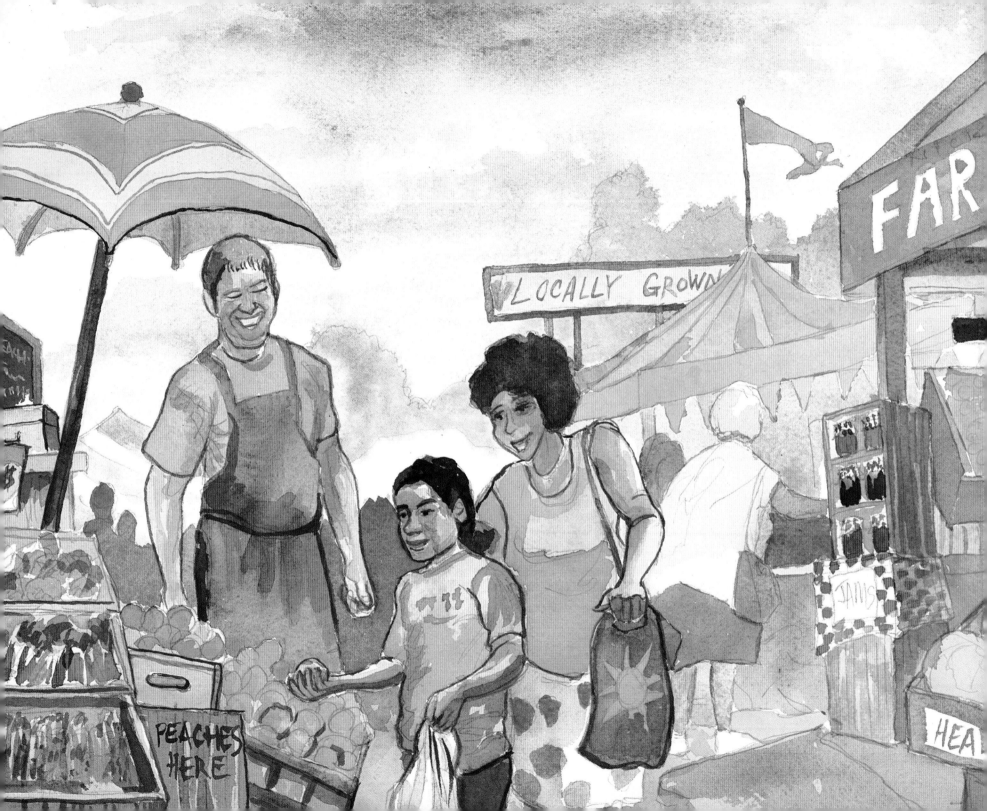

I express my feelings.

I squeal and dance with friends when we plan a sleepover. I turn to my coach for support when I'm feeling overwhelmed or frustrated. I show compassion when others are in need, brightening them up with jokes or warming them up with hugs.

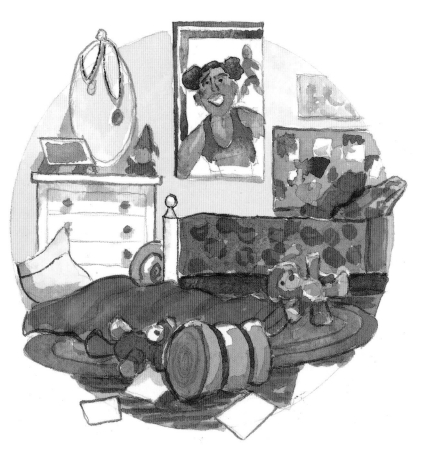

Expreso mis sentimientos.

Suelo bailar cuando planeamos una pijamada. Pido ayuda a mi entrenador cuando me siento abrumada o frustrada. Demuestro compasión hacia la gente que lo necesita alegrando sus días con una broma o confortándolos con un fuerte abrazo.

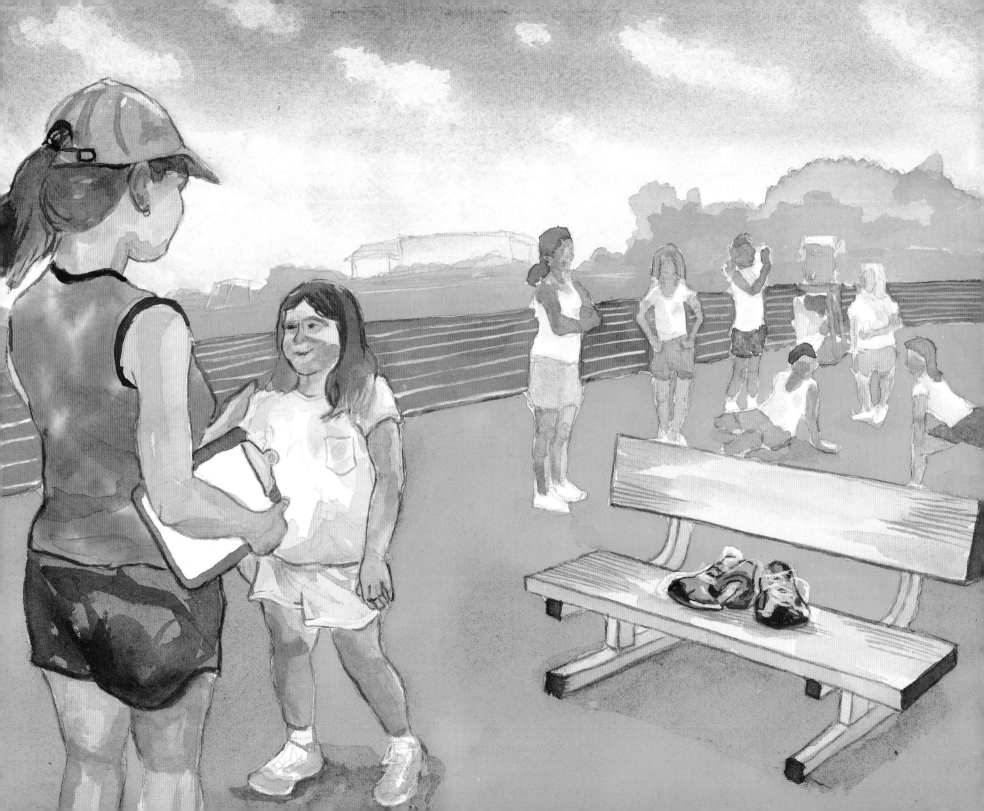

I am strong.

Soy fuerte.

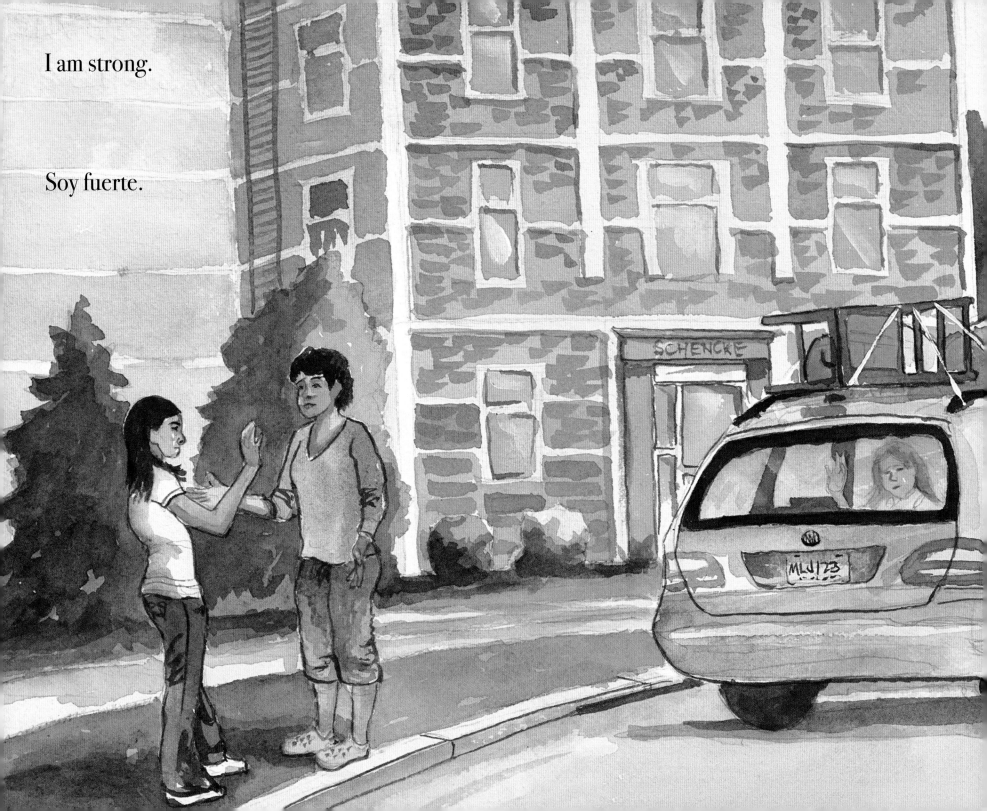

My body becomes more flexible as I run. My mind sharpens and my spirit soars. I offer help to younger children on the playground and ask for help when I don't understand a homework assignment. I let myself cry as I wave good-bye to a friend moving across the country.

Mi cuerpo se empieza a hacer más flexible cuando corro, mi mente se aclara y mi espíritu se eleva. Ofrezco ayuda a los niños más chicos cuando juegan en el parque y pido ayuda con mi tarea cuando no entiendo como hacerla. Permito a mis lágrimas rodar por mis mejillas mientras le digo adiós a un amigo que se muda a otra ciudad.

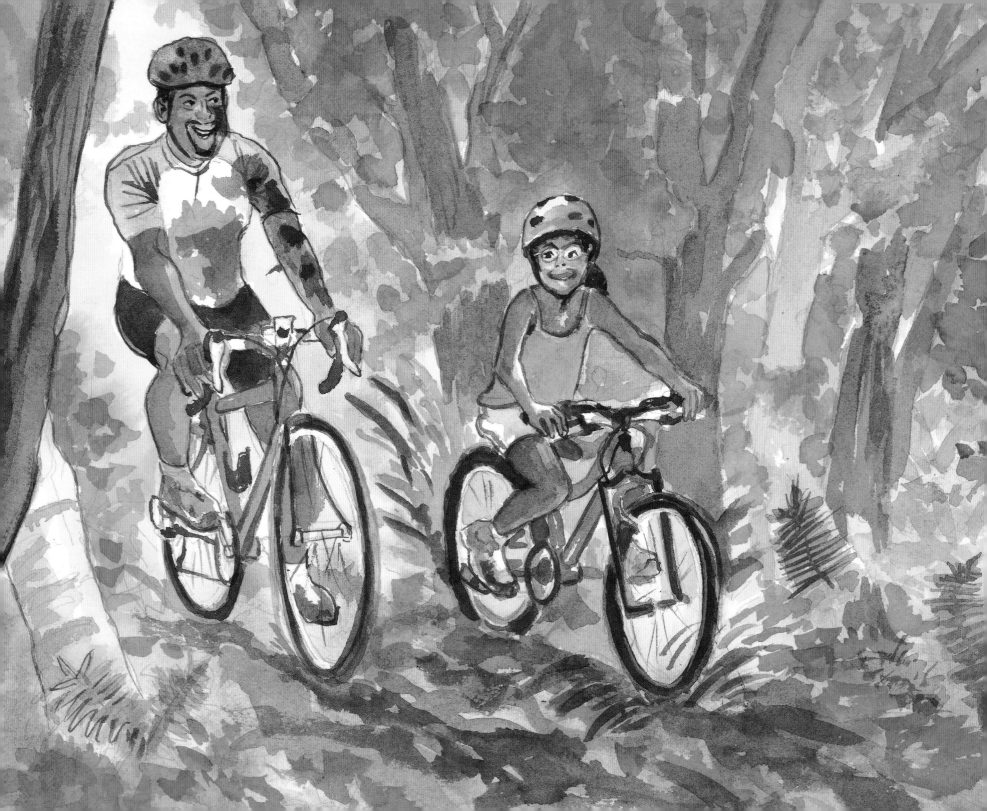

I am loveable.

I share my energy and talents with people around me. I can fly over a bush in a single bound as I play tag with my brothers and sisters in the yard. I splash mud up to my eyebrows as I pedal through a puddle on a bike ride with my dad. I have the patience to read my wiggly little cousin his favorite book for the thousandth time and the creativity to develop a secret cookie recipe.

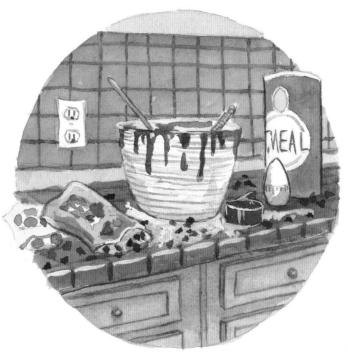

Soy adorable.

Comparto mi energía y talentos con las personas que me rodean. Puedo volar sobre los arbustos en un solo salto cuando juego con mis hermanos en el jardín al voto y me lleno de lodo hasta las cejas cuando pedaleo la bici a través de los charcos con mi papá. Tengo paciencia con mi pequeño sobrino cuando le leo sus cuentos favoritos por enésima vez y la creatividad para crear una receta secreta de galletas.

I have a positive attitude.

I record the best things about my day in a journal before I go to bed. I compliment my brother when he does well on his math tests and offer him encouragement when he struggles. I turn my chores into games, scrubbing the bathtub as if I'm a diver in an aquarium cleaning algae off the glass as exotic fish wriggle past.

Tengo una actitud positiva.

Escribo en mi diario las mejores cosas que me pasaron en el día antes de irme a la cama. Felicito a mi hermano cuando sale bien en los exámenes de matemáticas y lo estimulo para que siga esforzándose. Convierto mis tareas domésticas en juegos, cuando tallo mi bañera, me imagino que estoy zambullida en un acuario y estoy limpiando las algas del vidrio mientras una exótica variedad de peces pasa por mi lado.

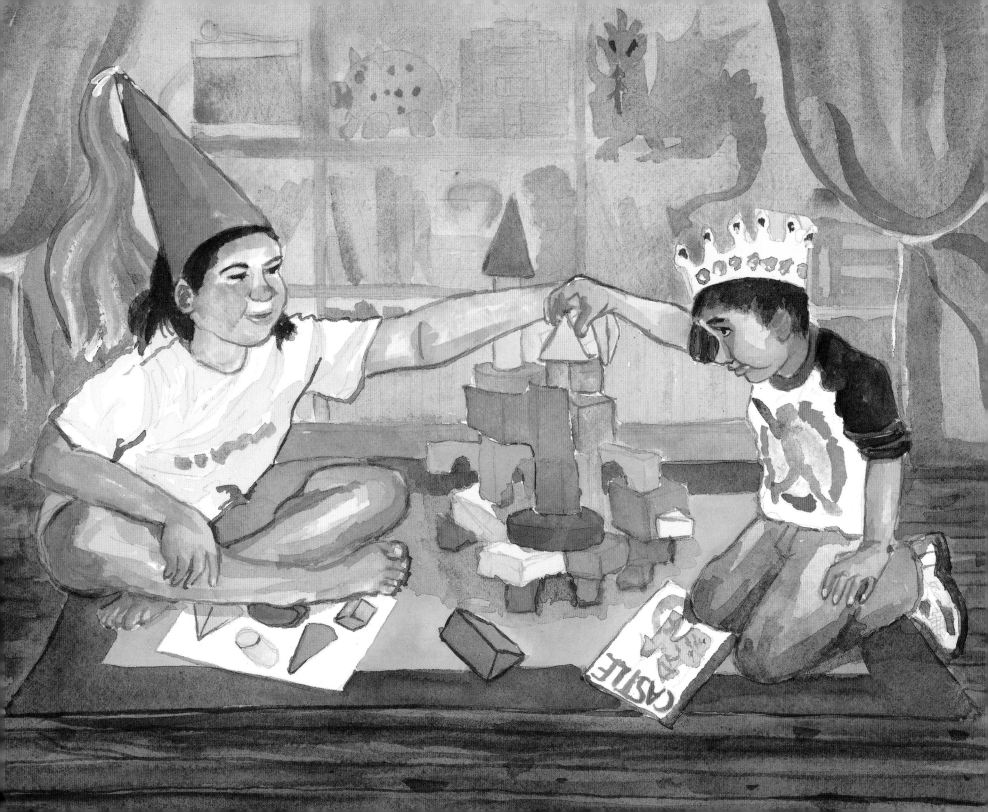

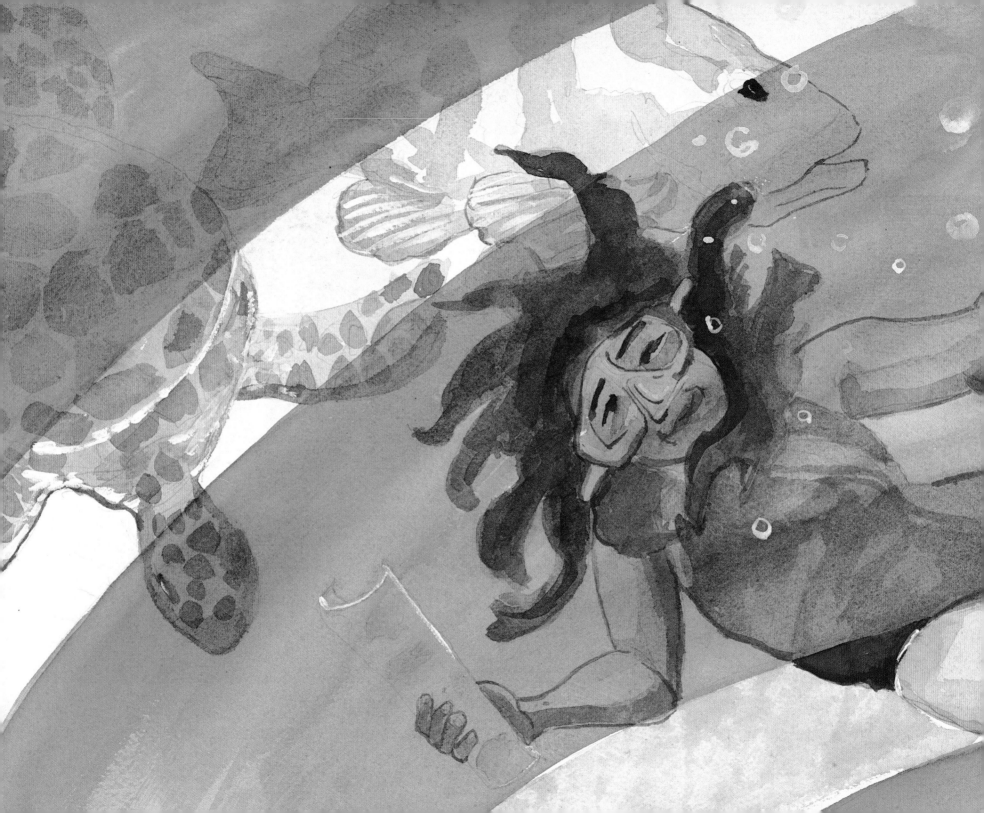

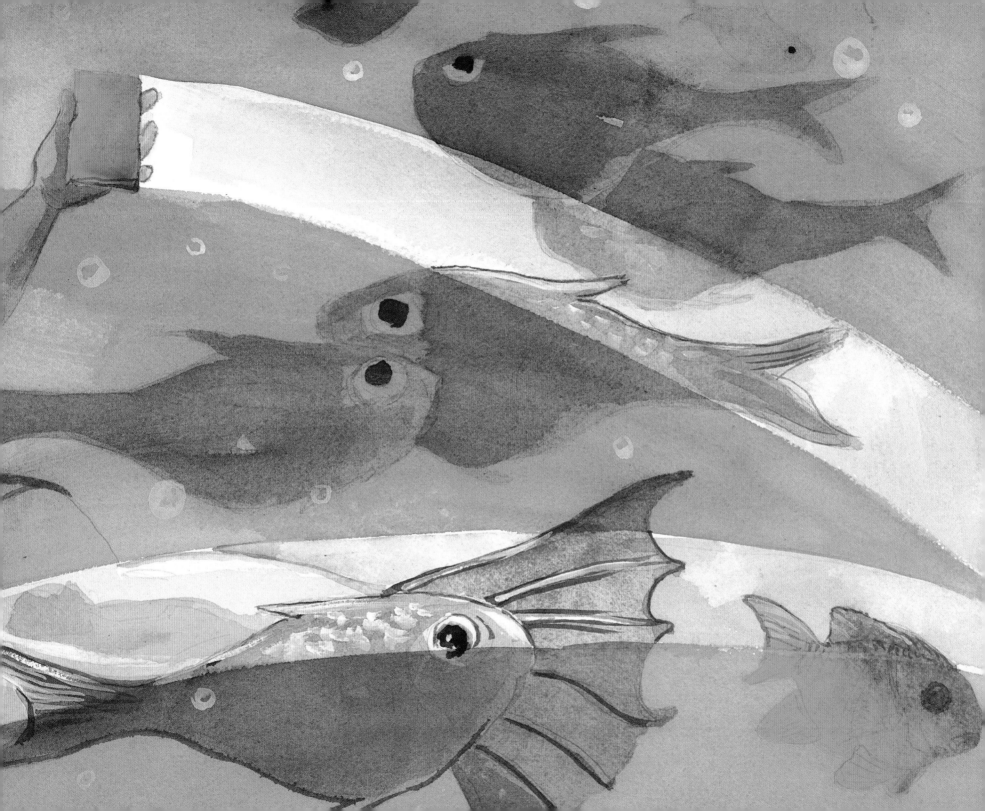

I am successful.

My dreams, numerous and beautiful, express my inner energy and passion. When I finish a race, my heart soars and I'm proud that I stayed true to my training and realized a dream. My fellow runners and I congratulate one another with high-fives and hugs and then excitedly begin planning our next challenge.

Soy exitosa.

Mis numerosos y hermosos sueños expresan mi energía y mi pasión interna. Cuando termino una carrera, mi corazón se eleva y me siento orgullosa de haberme mantenido apegada al entrenamiento para poder cumplir mi sueno. Mis compañeros de carrera y yo nos felicitamos unos a los otros con un choque de manos y abrazos y comenzamos emocionados a planear nuestro trabajo para el siguiente reto.

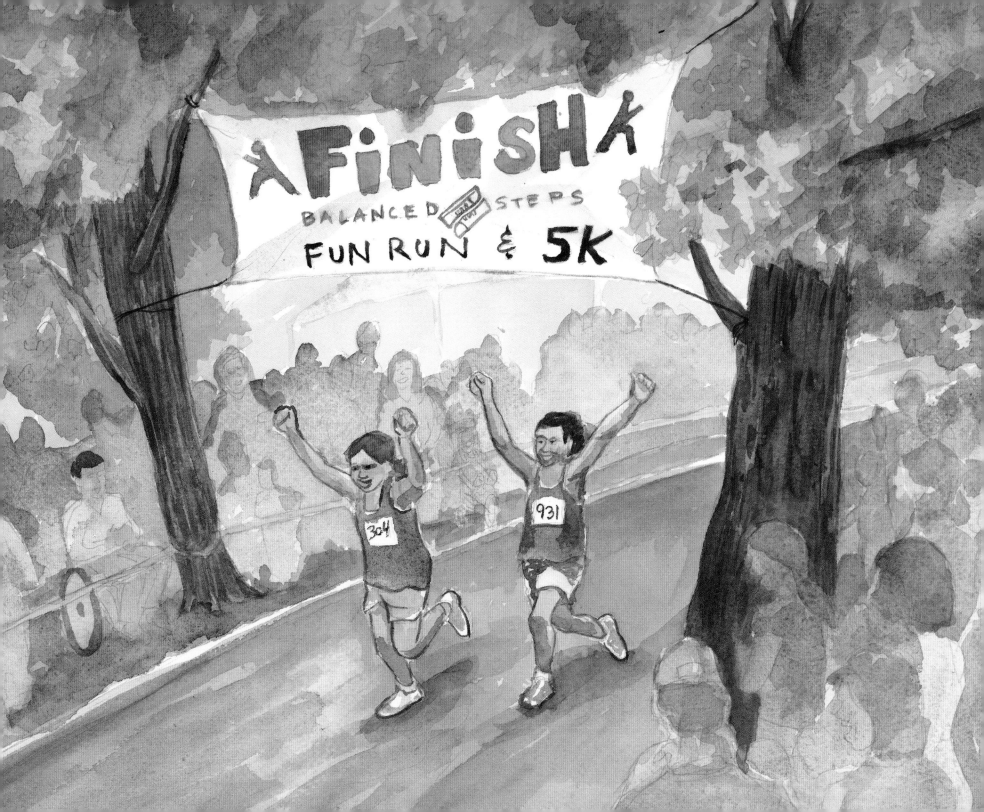

I am peaceful.

I stretch out in a soft, grassy area to gaze at clouds streaming across the sky. I pump my legs to soar high on a swing and relax to listen to the sounds around me. I walk silently beside a friend after we run, cooling down my body and relaxing my mind.

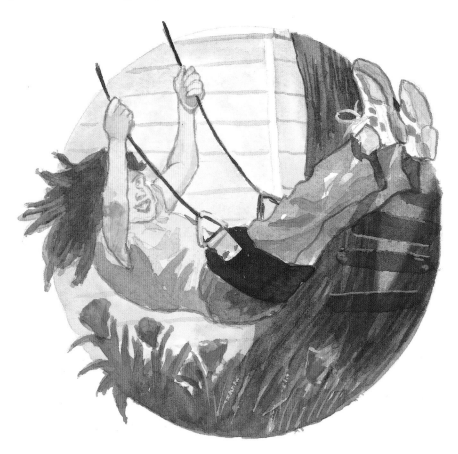

Soy tranquila.

Me estiro sobre un jardín suave para ver las nubes que fluyen a través del cielo. Levanto mis piernas muy alto en un bamboleo y me relajo escuchando los sonidos a mí alrededor. Camino silenciosamente al lado de mi amigo después de correr, relajando mi cuerpo y mi mente.

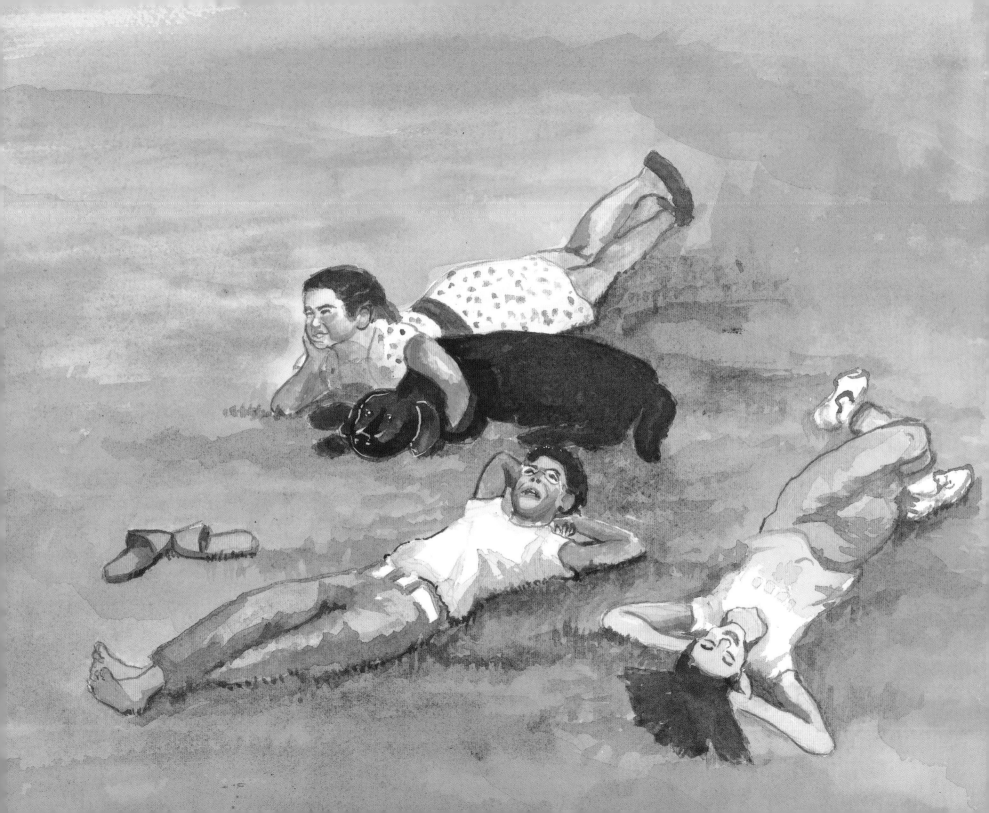

I like who I am.

Me gusta quien soy.

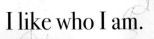

I am a vibrant girl who loves to giggle and feel the wind in my hair. I am a curious girl who likes to ask questions and discover how the world works. I am a confident girl, embracing my identity and loving life.

Soy una chica brillante que ama reír a carcajadas y sentir el viento sobre mi cabello. Soy una chica curiosa que le gusta hacer preguntas y descubrir como funciona el mundo. Soy una chica segura que adora quien es y ama la vida.

We are girls who love to run.

Somos chicas y a nosotras nos encanta correr.

"Running is fun because you can do it by yourself or with friends." – Maia, 6 1/2

"Running makes me feel tired but stronger after my hard work." – Maddie, 9

"Al coarrer me siento fuerte." – Amber 10

"My favorite thing about running is finishing the race because you have worked hard for something and have accomplished it." – Claire, 11

"I feel very refreshed and proud of myself when I'm finished." – Erin, 12

Al correr, me siento como puedo hacer cualqier cosa. – Angela, 12

"Running makes me feel good because I feel a sense of accomplishment toward my body." – Jessica, 13

"I enjoy running with my mother - it is something that we can do together." – Anna, 16

"Running makes me feel free and open, like I can truly connect with myself and my surroundings and relax." – Abby, 20

"Sometimes running makes me feel like a computer that is rebooting or a compass that is being re-oriented." – Ann, 43

"Physically running keeps me in great shape. Mentally and emotionally it keeps me balanced. Spiritually it keeps me centered." – Rhonnie, 51

"La mejor sensación que siento cuando corro, es que me hace sentir viva." – Jean, 53

"I like to race my grandchildren to see if I can win the race." – Mary Anne, 73

Author **Brianna K. Grant** is a girl who loves to run. She also keeps her creative juices flowing by writing special interest pieces for *The River Current News*, newsletter articles, and children's stories. Her teaching experience led Brianna to meet with Girls on the Run program founder Molly Barker.

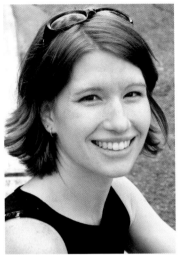

On a cloudy Seattle morning they discussed ideas that ultimately became *We Are Girls Who Love to Run*, fulfilling Brianna's life-long dream of writing a book. She earned her Bachelor's Degree in Art History from the University of Georgia and Master's in Teaching from Queens University of Charlotte. Brianna writes, runs, hikes, quilts and practices yoga in Duvall, Washington where she lives with her husband David, two children and dog.

• • •

Illustrator **Nicholas A. Wright** derives his artistic inspiration from the outdoors, especially the playgrounds of his youth, the Adirondack Mountains and St. Lawrence River. After winning a state-wide coloring contest when he was six, Nick dreamed of

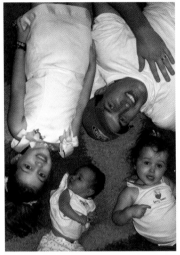

being an artist when he grew up. He graduated with a BFA from Ringling School of Art and Design in Sarasota, Florida and lives his dream as a monthly contributor to *Bow & Arrow Hunting Magazine* and full-time freelance artist. Nick illustrates paints, hunts and canoes in and around Glens Falls, New York where he lives with his wife Emily and three daughters, the youngest of which was born during the illustration of

We Are Girls Who Love to Run.

• • •

Autora **Brianna K. Grant** es una chica y a ella le encanta correr. También, cultiva su creatividad por escribir ensayos de interés especial para *The River Current News*, artículos para hojas informativas, y cuentos para niños. Sus experiencias de enseñar, la motivaron encontrarse con Molly Barker, la fundadora del programa <<Girls on the Run.>> En esta mañana nublada en Seattle, discutieron las ideas que llegaron a ser *Somos Chicas y A Nosotras Nos Encanta Correr*, realizando el sueño de Brianna de escribir un libro. Brianna ganó su Bachelors en la historia de arte de la Universidad de Georgia y su Maestría en Enseñar en La Universidad de Queens en Charlotte. Escribe, corre, va de excursión a pie, acolcha, y practica yoga en Duvall, Washington donde vive con su esposo, David, dos hijos y perro.

Ilustrador **Nicholas A. Wright** deriva su inspiración artística del aire libre, especialmente los campos de recreo de su juventud: Las Montañas de los Adirondacks y el Río de St. Lawrence. Después de ganar un concurso de colorar por todo el estado cuando tenía seis años, Nick sonaba con ser artista al crecer. Se graduó con un BFA de la Universidad de Ringling de Arte y Diseño en Sarasota, Florida y realiza su sueño al contribuir cada mes a *Bow & Arrow Hunting Magazine* y es un artista autónomo tiempo completo. Nick dibuja, pinta, caza y va en canoa en y alrededor de las Caídas de Glens, Nueva York donde vive con su esposa, Emily, y sus tres hijas. La menor nació mientras Nick trabajaba en *Somos Chicas y A Nosotras Nos Encanta Correr*.